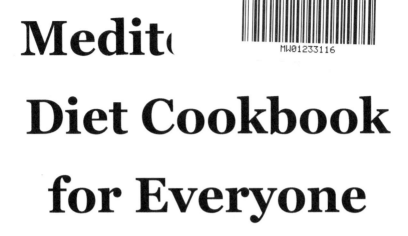

Medit‹

Diet Cookbook

for Everyone

Find the Perfect Balance
with 50 Healthy and Tasty
Recipes

By Tracey Lane

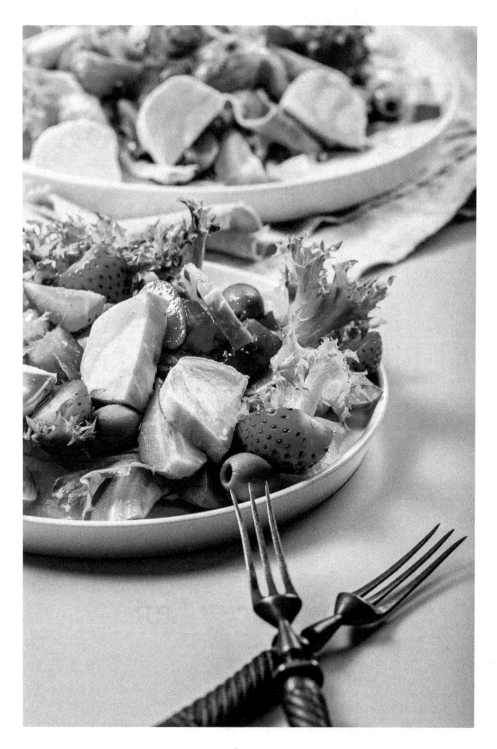

Table of Contents

Introduction

Mediterranean diet is based on the eating habits of the inhabitants of the regions along the Mediterranean Sea, mostly from Italy, Spain and Greece; it is considered more a life style then a diet, in fact it also promotes physical activity and proper liquid (mostly water) consumption.

Depending on fresh seasonal local foods there are no strict rules, because of the many cultural differences, but there are some common factors.

Mediterranean diet has become famous for its ability to reduce heart disease and obesity, thanks to the low consumption of unhealthy fats that increase blood glucose.

Mediterranean diet is mostly plant based, so it's rich of antioxidants; vegetables, fruits like apple and grapes, olive oil, whole grains, herbs, beans and nuts are consumed in large quantities.

Moderate amounts of poultry, eggs, dairy and seafood are also common aliments, accompanied by a little bit of red wine (some studies say that in small amount it helps to stay healthy).

Red meat and sweets like cookies and cakes are accepted but are more limited in quantity.

Foods to avoid:

- refined grains, such as white bread and pasta
- dough containing white flour refined oils (even canola oil and soybean oil)
- foods with added sugars (like pastries, sodas, and candies)
- processed meats processed or packaged foods

Chapter 1: Breakfast and Snack Recipes

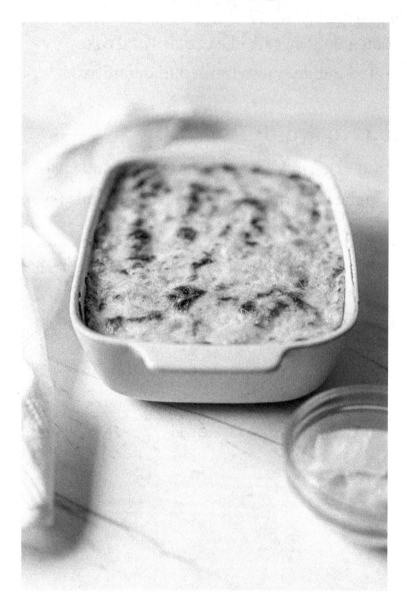

Mango and Spinach Bowls

Servings: 4 | Cooking: 0 min

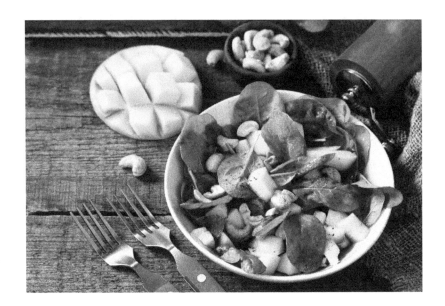

Ingredients

- 1 cup baby arugula
- 1 cup baby spinach, chopped
- 1 mango, peeled and cubed
- 1 cup strawberries, halved
- 1 tablespoon hemp seeds
- 1 cucumber, sliced
- 1 tablespoon lime juice
- 1 tablespoon tahini paste

- 1 tablespoon water

Directions

1. In a salad bowl, mix the arugula with the rest of the ingredients except the tahini and the water and toss.
2. In a small bowl, combine the tahini with the water, whisk well, add to the salad, toss, divide into small bowls and serve for breakfast.

Nutrition: calories 211; fat 4.5; fiber 6.5; carbs 10.2; protein 3.5

Veggie Quiche

Servings: 8 | Cooking: 55 min

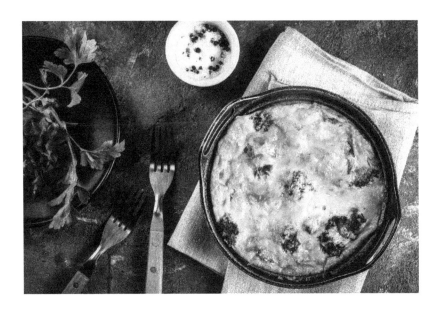

Ingredients

- ½ cup sun-dried tomatoes, chopped
- 1 prepared pie crust
- 2 tablespoons avocado oil
- 1 yellow onion, chopped
- 2 garlic cloves, minced
- 2 cups spinach, chopped
- 1 red bell pepper, chopped
- ¼ cup kalamata olives, pitted and sliced

- 1 teaspoon parsley flakes
- 1 teaspoon oregano, dried
- 1/3 cup feta cheese, crumbled
- 4 eggs, whisked
- 1 and ½ cups almond milk
- 1 cup cheddar cheese, shredded
- Salt and black pepper to the taste

Directions

1. Heat up a pan with the oil over medium-high heat, add the garlic and onion and sauté for 3 minutes.
2. Add the bell pepper and sauté for 3 minutes more.
3. Add the olives, parsley, spinach, oregano, salt and pepper and cook everything for 5 minutes.
4. Add tomatoes and the cheese, toss and take off the heat.
5. Arrange the pie crust in a pie plate, pour the spinach and tomatoes mix inside and spread.
6. In a bowl, mix the eggs with salt, pepper, the milk and half of the cheese, whisk and pour over the mixture in the pie crust.
7. Sprinkle the remaining cheese on top and bake at 375 degrees F for 40 minutes.

8. Cool the quiche down, slice and serve for breakfast.

Nutrition: calories 211; fat 14.4; fiber 1.4; carbs 12.5; protein 8.6

Tuna and Cheese Bake

Servings: 4 | Cooking: 15 min

Ingredients

- 10 ounces canned tuna, drained and flaked
- 4 eggs, whisked
- ½ cup feta cheese, shredded
- 1 tablespoon chives, chopped
- 1 tablespoon parsley, chopped
- Salt and black pepper to the taste
- 3 teaspoons olive oil

Directions

1. Grease a baking dish with the oil, add the tuna and the rest of the ingredients except the cheese, toss and bake at 370 degrees F for 15 minutes.
2. Sprinkle the cheese on top, leave the mix aside for 5 minutes, slice and serve for breakfast.

Nutrition: calories 283; fat 14.2; fiber 5.6; carbs 12.1; protein 6.4

Tomato and Cucumber Salad

Servings: 4 | Cooking: 5 min

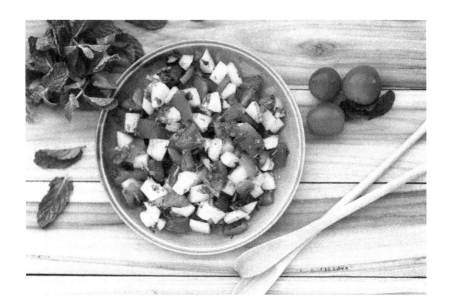

Ingredients

- 3 tomatoes, chopped
- 2 cucumbers, chopped
- 1 red onion, sliced
- 2 red bell peppers, chopped
- ¼ cup fresh cilantro, chopped
- 1 tablespoon capers
- 1 oz whole-grain bread, chopped
- 1 tablespoon canola oil

- ½ teaspoon minced garlic
- 1 tablespoon Dijon mustard
- 1 teaspoon olive oil
- 1 teaspoon lime juice

Directions

1. Pour canola oil in the skillet and bring it to boil.
2. Add chopped bread and roast it until crunchy (3-5 minutes).
3. Meanwhile, in the salad bowl combine together sliced red onion, cucumbers, tomatoes, bell peppers, cilantro, capers, and mix up gently.
4. Make the dressing: mix up together lime juice, olive oil, Dijon mustard, and minced garlic.
5. Pour the dressing over the salad and stir it directly before serving.

Nutrition: calories 136; fat 5.7; fiber 4.1; carbs 20.2; protein 4.1

Cream Olive Muffins

Servings: 6 | Cooking: 20 min

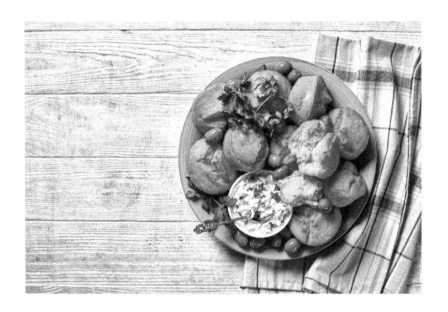

Ingredients

- ½ cup quinoa, cooked
- 2 oz Feta cheese, crumbled
- 2 eggs, beaten
- 3 kalamata olives, chopped
- ¾ cup heavy cream
- 1 tomato, chopped
- 1 teaspoon butter, softened
- 1 tablespoon wheat flour, whole grain

- ½ teaspoon salt

Directions

1. In the mixing bowl whisk eggs and add Feta cheese.
2. Then add chopped tomato and heavy cream.
3. After this, add wheat flour, salt, and quinoa.
4. Then add kalamata olives and mix up the ingredients with the help of the spoon.
5. Brush the muffin molds with the butter from inside.
6. Transfer quinoa mixture in the muffin molds and flatten it with the help of the spatula or spoon if needed.
7. Cook the muffins in the preheated to 355F oven for 20 minutes.

Nutrition: calories 165; fat 10.8; fiber 1.2; carbs 11.5; protein 5.8

Roasted Asparagus with Prosciutto and Poached Egg

Servings: 4 | Cooking: 25 min

Ingredients

- 1 bunch fresh asparagus, trimmed
- 1 tablespoon extra-virgin olive oil
- 4 eggs
- 2 ounces minced prosciutto
- 1/2 lemon, zested and juiced
- 1 tablespoon olive oil
- 1 pinch salt
- 1 pinch ground black pepper
- 1 teaspoon distilled white vinegar
- Ground black pepper

Directions

1. Preheat oven to 425F or 220C.
2. In a baking dish, place the asparagus and drizzle with the extra-virgin olive oil.
3. In a skillet, heat the olive oil over medium-low heat; add the prosciutto and cook for about 3-4 minutes, stirring, until golden and rendered.

Sprinkle over the asparagus in the baking dish and season with black pepper; toss to coat.

4. Roast for 10 minutes, toss, return to the oven, and continue roasting for 5 minutes or until the asparagus are tender yet firm to the bite.

5. Fill a large saucepan with about 2-3 inches of water; bring to a boil over high heat. When boiling, reduce the heat to low; pour in the vinegar and a pinch of salt. Crack an egg into a small bowl, then gently slip the egg into the water. Repeat with the remaining eggs. Poach the eggs for about 4-6 minutes or until the whites are firm and the yolks are thick but not hard. With a slotted spoon, remove the eggs, dab the scoop on a clean kitchen towel to remove excess water from the eggs, and transfer to a warm plate.

6. Drizzle the asparagus with the lemon juice and transfer divide between 2 plates. Top each asparagus bed with the 2 poached eggs, sprinkle with a pinch of lemon zest, and season with black pepper; serve.

Nutrition:163 Cal, 12.3 g total fat (2.7 g sat. fat), 171 mg chol., 273 mg sodium, 4.3 g carb., 1.9 g fiber, 10.4 g protein.

Figs Oatmeal

Servings: 5 | Cooking: 20 min

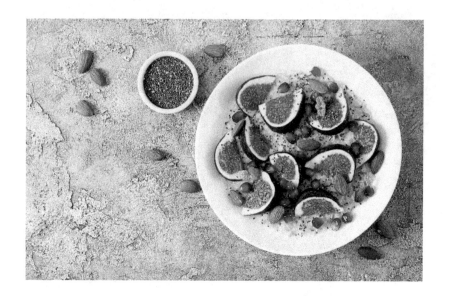

Ingredients

- 2 cups oatmeal
- 1 ½ cup milk
- 1 tablespoon butter
- 3 figs, chopped
- 1 tablespoon honey

Directions

1. Pour milk in the saucepan.
2. Add oatmeal and close the lid.

3. Cook the oatmeal for 15 minutes over the medium-low heat.
4. Then add chopped figs and honey.
5. Add butter and mix up the oatmeal well.
6. Cook it for 5 minutes more.
7. Close the lid and let the cooked breakfast rest for 10 minutes before serving.

Nutrition: calories 222; fat 6; fiber 4.4; carbs 36.5; protein 7.1

Mediterranean Freezer Breakfast Wraps

Servings: 4 | Cooking: 3 min

Ingredients

- 1 cup spinach leaves, fresh, chopped
- 1 tablespoon water or low-fat milk
- 1/2 teaspoon garlic-chipotle seasoning or your preferred seasoning
- 4 eggs, beaten
- 4 pieces (8-inch) whole-wheat tortillas
- 4 tablespoons tomato chutney (or dried tomatoes, chopped or canned tomatoes)
- 4 tablespoons feta cheese, crumbled (or goat cheese)
- Optional: prosciutto, chopped or bacon, cooked, crumbled
- Salt and pepper, to taste

Directions

1. In a mixing bowl, whisk the eggs, water or milk, and seasoning together.

26

2. Heat a skillet with a bit of olive oil; pour the eggs and scramble for about 3-4 minutes, or until just cooked.
3. Lay the tortillas in a clean surface; divide the eggs between them, arranging the scrambled eggs in a line and leaving the tortilla edges free to fold later.
4. Top the egg layer with about 1 tablespoon of cheese, 1 tablespoon tomatoes, and 1/4 cup spinach. If using, layer with prosciutto or bacon.
5. In a burrito-style, roll up the tortillas, folding both of the ends in the process.
6. In a panini maker or a clean skillet, cook for about 1 minute, turning once, until the tortilla wraps are crisp and brown; serve.

Nutrition:450 Cal, 15 g total fat (5 g sat. fat), 220 mg chol., 1, 280 mg sodium, 960 mg pot., 64 g carb.,6 g fiber,20 g sugar, 17 g protein.

Cheesy Olives Bread

Servings: 10 | Cooking: 30 min

Ingredients

- 4 cups whole-wheat flour
- 3 tablespoons oregano, chopped
- 2 teaspoons dry yeast
- ¼ cup olive oil
- 1 and ½ cups black olives, pitted and sliced
- 1 cup water
- ½ cup feta cheese, crumbled

Directions

1. In a bowl, mix the flour with the water, the yeast and the oil, stir and knead your dough very well.
2. Put the dough in a bowl, cover with plastic wrap and keep in a warm place for 1 hour.
3. Divide the dough into 2 bowls and stretch each ball really well.
4. Add the rest of the ingredients on each ball and tuck them inside well kneading the dough again.
5. Flatten the balls a bit and leave them aside for 40 minutes more.

6. Transfer the balls to a baking sheet lined with parchment paper, make a small slit in each and bake at 425 degrees F for 30 minutes.
7. Serve the bread as a Mediterranean breakfast.

Nutrition: calories 251; fat 7.3; fiber 2.1; carbs 39.7; protein 6.7

Scrambled Eggs

Servings: 2 | Cooking: 10 min

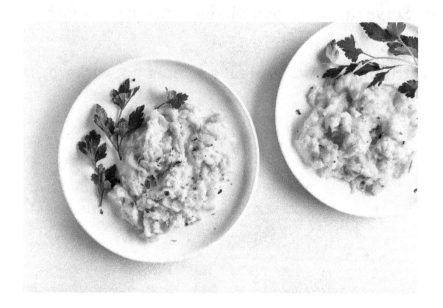

Ingredients

- 1 yellow bell pepper, chopped
- 8 cherry tomatoes, cubed
- 2 spring onions, chopped
- 1 tablespoon olive oil
- 1 tablespoon capers, drained
- 2 tablespoons black olives, pitted and sliced
- 4 eggs
- A pinch of salt and black pepper

- ¼ teaspoon oregano, dried
- 1 tablespoon parsley, chopped

Directions

1. Heat up a pan with the oil over medium-high heat, add the bell pepper and spring onions and sauté for 3 minutes.
2. Add the tomatoes, capers and the olives and sauté for 2 minutes more.
3. Crack the eggs into the pan, add salt, pepper and the oregano and scramble for 5 minutes more.
4. Divide the scramble between plates, sprinkle the parsley on top and serve.

Nutrition: calories 249; fat 17; fiber 3.2; carbs 13.3; protein 13.5

Chapter 2: Lunch & Dinner Recipes

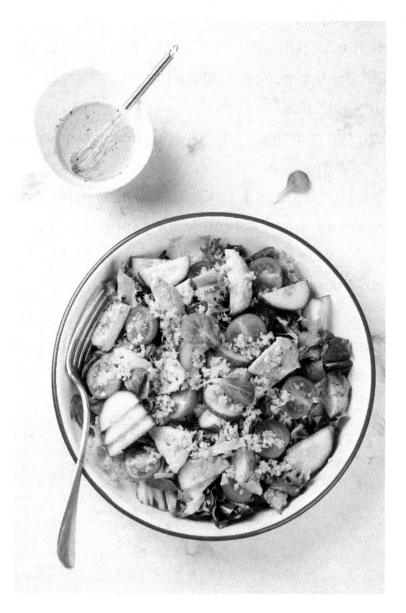

Broccoli, Chicken, and Quinoa Salad with Roasted Lemon Dressing

Servings: 4 | Kcal per serving: 481

Ingredients

- 1/2 cup fresh mint (chopped)
- 1/2 cup dried cranberries
- 3/4 cup toasted chopped walnuts
- 2 cups arugula
- 1 tablespoon Dijon mustard
- 1/4 cup red wine vinegar
- 1 medium broccoli (with stems)
- 1/2 cup quinoa
- 1 cup chicken broth (low-sodium)
- 2 lemons (deseeded and thinly sliced)
- 1/8 teaspoon, plus 1/4 teaspoon salt (divided)
- 4 tablespoons extra-virgin olive oil (divided)
- 8 ounces chicken breast (skinless, boneless, trimmed)

Directions

1. Place meat on one side of a baking sheet and top with a tablespoon of oil and 1/8 teaspoon salt. Roast for 10 min in a preheated oven at 425 degrees.

2. Put the lemon slices on the other side of the baking sheet. Roast until browned while flipping them once.

3. Put quinoa and broth in a saucepan over medium-high flame, and bring to a boil. Reduce flame settings and cover the pan. Cook on low flame until most of the liquid is absorbed or about 15 min. Turn off the heat and rest for 10 min.

4. Cut the broccoli florets into bite-size pieces. Slice and chop the stems.

5. Transfer half of the roasted lemon slices to a chopping board and chop. Place in a bowl, and add 1/4 teaspoon salt, 3 tablespoons oil, mustard, and vinegar. Mix well.

6. Place the roasted meat on a chopping board and shred. Place in a bowl, and add mint, cranberries, walnuts, arugula, cooked quinoa, broccoli, and the rest of the lemon slices. Add the dressing, and gently toss until combined.

Tasty Greek Pasta

Servings: 4 | Kcal per serving: 487

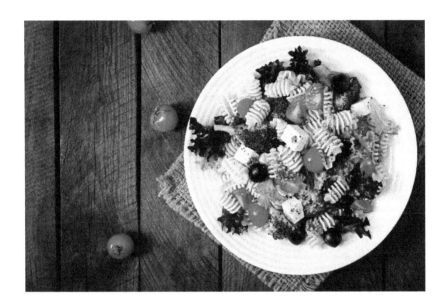

Ingredients

- 1/2 cup crumbled feta cheese
- 1/4 cup pitted Kalamata olives (chopped)
- 6 cups whole-wheat rotini pasta (cooked)
- Chopped fresh basil for serving
- 4 cups baby spinach (lightly packed)
- 1 8-ounce can tomato salt (no salt added)
- 1 garlic clove (minced)
- 1 cup minced onion

- 9 ounces chicken sausage or 3 links (cooked and sliced)
- 2 tablespoons olive oil

Directions

1. Preheat a skillet on a medium-high flame. Add oil, and cook the garlic, onion, and sausage for 6 min while stirring often.
2. Add olives, pasta, spinach, and tomato sauce. Cook for 5 more min while frequently stirring to make sure that the pasta won't stick to the pan.
3. You can stir in up to 2 tablespoons of water if necessary.
4. Stir in basil and feta, remove from heat, and serve.

Sweet Potato Stuffing Served with Hummus Dressing

Servings: 1 | Kcal per serving: 472

Ingredients

- 1 tablespoon water
- 1/4 cup hummus
- 1 cup black beans (rinsed and drained)
- 3/4 cup chopped kale (rinsed and drained)
- 1 big sweet potato (scrubbed)

Directions

1. Use a fork to prick the potato. Cook in the microwave at a high temperature setting up to 10 min.
2. Put kale in a pan over medium-high flame. Cover and cook until wilted while stirring twice during the process. Add up to 2 tablespoons of water and beans. Cook for a couple of min or until steaming hot.
3. Divide the sweet potato and place it on a plate. Top with the bean and kale mixture.

4. Put 2 tablespoons of water in a small bowl. Add the hummus and mix until combined. You can add more water until you get your preferred consistency. Drizzle sauce on top of the potato and beans.

Lemon, Buttered Shrimp Panini

Preparation: 9 min | Cooking: 8 min | Servings: 4

Ingredient

- 3 tbsp. butter
- 1 baguette
- 1 tsp hot sauce
- 1 tbsp. parsley
- 2 tbsp. lemon juice
- 4 garlic cloves, minced
- 1 lb. shrimp peeled

Directions:

1. Make a hollowed portion on your baguette. Sauté the following on a skillet with melted butter: parsley, hot sauce, lemon juice and garlic. After 3 min, mix in the shrimps and sautéing for five min.
2. Scoop shrimps into baguette and grill in a Panini press until baguette is crisped and ridged.

Nutrition: Calories: 262; Protein: 26.1g; Fat: 10.8g

Sun-Dried Tomatoes Panini

Preparation: 6 min | Cooking: 16 min | Servings: 4

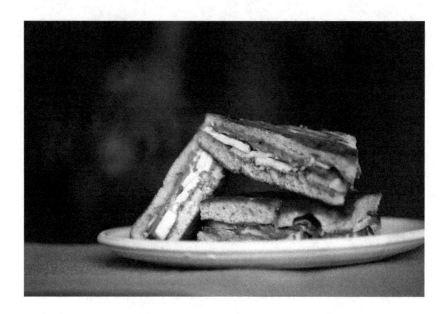

Ingredient

- ½ cup shredded mozzarella cheese
- 8 slices country style Italian bread
- 1/8 tsp freshly ground black pepper
- Cooking spray
- 3/8 tsp salt, divided
- 1 6oz package fresh baby spinach
- 8 garlic cloves, thinly sliced
- 1/8 tsp crushed red pepper

- ¼ cup chopped drained oil packed sun-dried tomato
- 4 4oz chicken cutlets
- 1 tsp chopped rosemary
- 2 tbsp. extra virgin olive oil, divided

Directions:

1. In a re-sealable bag mix chicken, rosemary and 2 tsp olive oil. Marinate for 35 min in the ref. On medium high fire, place a skillet and heat 4 tsp oil. Sauté for a minute garlic, red pepper and sun-dried tomato.

2. Add 1/8 tsp salt and spinach and cook for a minute and put aside. Using grill pan coated with cooking spray, grill chicken for three min per side. Season with black pepper and salt. To assemble the sandwich, evenly layer the following on one bread slice: cheese, spinach mixture, and chicken cutlet.

3. Cover with another bread slice. Situate sandwich in a Panini press and grill for around five min or until cheese is melted and bread is crisped and ridged.

Nutrition: Calories: 369; Protein: 42.7g; Fat: 10.1g

Chapter 3: Meat Recipes

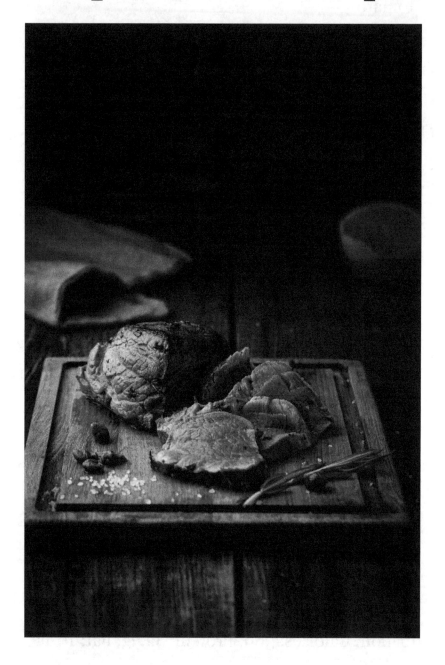

Peas And Ham Thick Soup

Servings: 4 | Cooking: 30 min

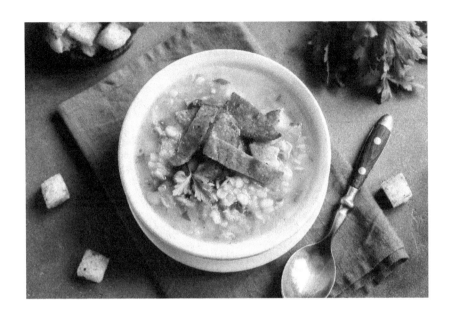

Ingredients

- Pepper and salt to taste
- 1 lb. ham, coarsely chopped
- 24 oz frozen sweet peas
- 4 cup ham stock
- ¼ cup white wine
- 1 carrot, chopped coarsely
- 1 onion, chopped coarsely
- 2 tbsp butter, divided

Directions

1. On medium fireplace a medium pot and heat oil. Sauté for 6 minutes the onion or until soft and translucent.
2. Add wine and cook for 4 minutes or until nearly evaporated.
3. Add ham stock and bring to a simmer and simmer continuously while covered for 4 minutes.
4. Add peas and cook for 7 minutes or until tender.
5. Meanwhile, in a nonstick fry pan, cook to a browned crisp the ham in 1 tbsp butter, around 6 minutes. Remove from fire and set aside.
6. When peas are soft, transfer to a blender and puree. Return to pot, continue cooking while seasoning with pepper, salt and ½ of crisped ham. Once soup is to your desired taste, turn off fire.
7. Transfer to 4 serving bowls and garnish evenly with crisped ham.

Nutrition: Calories: 403; Carbs: 32.5g; Protein: 37.3g; Fat: 12.5g

Bell Peppers On Chicken Breasts

Servings: 6 | Cooking: 30 min

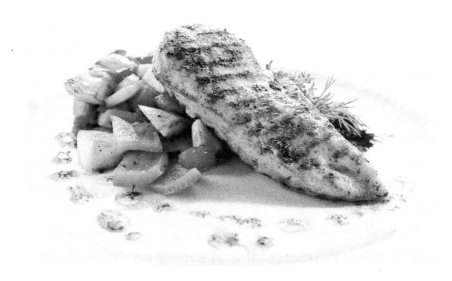

Ingredients

- ¼ tsp freshly ground black pepper
- ½ tsp salt
- 1 large red bell pepper, cut into ¼-inch strips
- 1 large yellow bell pepper, cut into ¼-inch strips
- 1 tbsp olive oil
- 1 tsp chopped fresh oregano
- 2 1/3 cups coarsely chopped tomato
- 2 tbsp finely chopped fresh flat-leaf parsley

- 20 Kalamata olives
- 3 cups onion sliced crosswise
- 6 4-oz skinless, boneless chicken breast halves, cut in half horizontally
- Cooking spray

Directions

1. On medium high fire, place a large nonstick fry pan and heat oil. Once oil is hot, sauté onions until soft and translucent, around 6 to 8 minutes.
2. Add bell peppers and sauté for another 10 minutes or until tender.
3. Add black pepper, salt and tomato. Cook until tomato juice has evaporated, around 7 minutes.
4. Add olives, oregano and parsley, cook until heated through around 1 to 2 minutes. Transfer to a bowl and keep warm.
5. Wipe pan with paper towel and grease with cooking spray. Return to fire and place chicken breasts. Cook for three minutes per side or until desired doneness is reached. If needed, cook chicken in batches.
6. When cooking the last batch of chicken is done, add back the previous batch of chicken and the

onion-bell pepper mixture and cook for a minute or two while tossing chicken to coat well in the onion-bell pepper mixture.

7. Serve and enjoy.

Nutrition: Calories: 261.8; Carbs: 11.0g; Protein: 36.0g; Fat: 8.2g

Yummy Turkey Meatballs

Servings: 4 | Cooking: 25 min

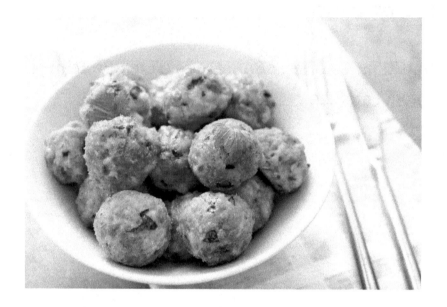

Ingredients

- ¼ yellow onion, finely diced
- 1 14-oz can of artichoke hearts, diced
- 1 lb. ground turkey
- 1 tsp dried parsley
- 1 tsp oil
- 4 tbsp fresh basil, finely chopped
- Pepper and salt to taste

Directions

1. Grease a cookie sheet and preheat oven to 3500F.
2. On medium fire, place a nonstick medium saucepan and sauté artichoke hearts and diced onions for 5 minutes or until onions are soft.
3. Remove from fire and let cool.
4. Meanwhile, in a big bowl, mix with hands parsley, basil and ground turkey. Season to taste.
5. Once onion mixture has cooled add into the bowl and mix thoroughly.
6. With an ice cream scooper, scoop ground turkey and form into balls, makes around 6 balls.
7. Place on prepped cookie sheet, pop in the oven and bake until cooked through around 15-20 minutes.
8. Remove from pan, serve and enjoy.

Nutrition: Calories: 328; Carbs: 11.8g; Protein: 33.5g; Fat: 16.3g

Garlic Caper Beef Roast

Servings: 4 | Cooking: 40 min

Ingredients

- 2 lbs beef roast, cubed
- 1 tbsp fresh parsley, chopped
- 1 tbsp capers, chopped
- 1 tbsp garlic, minced
- 1 cup chicken stock
- 1/2 tsp dried rosemary
- 1/2 tsp ground cumin
- 1 onion, chopped
- 1 tbsp olive oil
- Pepper
- Salt

Directions

1. Add oil into the instant pot and set the pot on sauté mode.
2. Add garlic and onion and sauté for 5 minutes.
3. Add meat and cook until brown.
4. Add remaining ingredients and stir well.

5. Seal pot with lid and cook on high for 30 minutes.
6. Once done, allow to release pressure naturally. Remove lid.
7. Stir well and serve.

Nutrition: Calories 470 Fat 17.9 g Carbohydrates 3.9 g Sugar 1.4 g Protein 69.5 g Cholesterol 203 mg

Olive Oil Drenched Lemon Chicken

Servings: 4 | Cooking: 60 min

Ingredients

- 1 lemon, thinly sliced
- 1 red bell pepper, cut into 1-inch wide strips
- 1 red onion, cut into 1-inch wedges
- 1 tablespoon dried oregano
- 1/2 teaspoon coarsely ground black pepper
- 1/4 cup olive oil
- 2 tablespoons fresh lemon juice
- 2 tablespoons fresh lemon zest
- 3/4 teaspoon salt
- 4 large cloves garlic, pressed
- 4 skinless, boneless chicken breast halves
- 8 baby red potatoes, halved

Directions

1. Preheat oven to 400oF.
2. In a bowl, mix well pepper, salt, oregano, garlic, lemon zest, lemon juice, and olive oil.

3. In a 9 x 13-inch casserole dish, evenly spread chicken in a single layer. Brush lemon juice mixture over chicken.
4. In a bowl mix well lemon slices, red onion, bell pepper, and potatoes. Drizzle remaining olive oil sauce and toss well to coat. Arrange vegetables and lemon slices around chicken breasts in baking dish.
5. Bake for 50 minutes; brush chicken and vegetables with pan drippings halfway through cooking time.
6. Let chicken rest for ten minutes before serving.

Nutrition: Calories: 517; Carbs: 65.1g; Protein: 30.8g; Fats: 16.7g

Chapter 4: Poultry Recipes

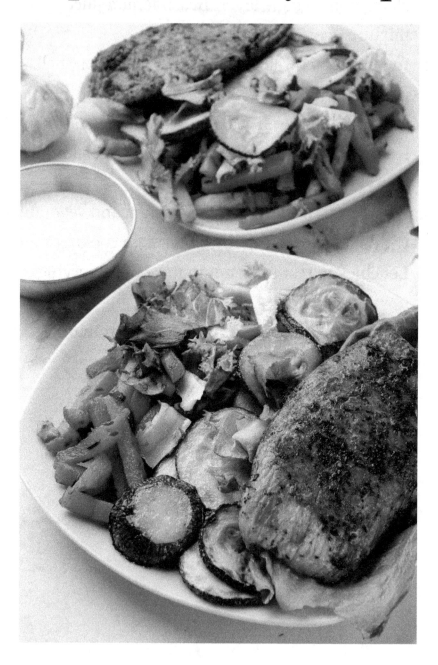

Chicken Wrap

Servings: 2 | Cooking: 0 min

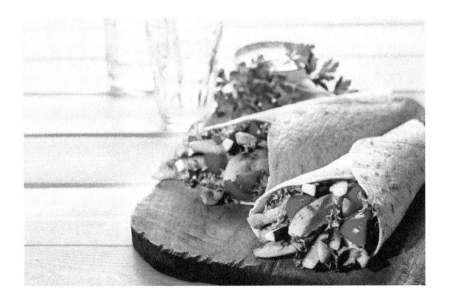

Ingredients

- 2 whole wheat tortilla flatbreads
- 6 chicken breast slices, skinless, boneless, cooked and shredded
- A handful baby spinach
- 2 provolone cheese slices
- 4 tomato slices
- 10 kalamata olives, pitted and sliced
- 1 red onion, sliced

- 2 tablespoons roasted peppers, chopped

Directions

1. Arrange the tortillas on a working surface, and divide the chicken and the other ingredients on each.
2. Roll the tortillas and serve them right away.

Nutrition: calories 190; fat 6.8; fiber 3.5; carbs 15.1; protein 6.6

Carrots And Tomatoes Chicken

Servings: 4 | Cooking: 1 Hour And 10 min

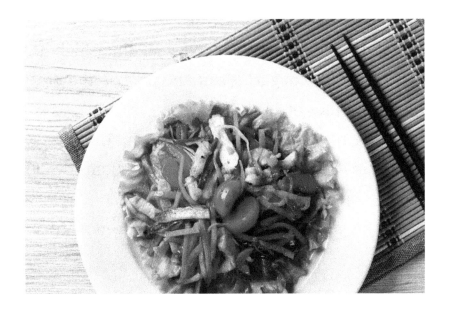

Ingredients

- 2 pounds chicken breasts, skinless, boneless and halved
- Salt and black pepper to the taste
- 3 garlic cloves, minced
- 3 tablespoons avocado oil
- 2 shallots, chopped
- 4 carrots, sliced
- 3 tomatoes, chopped

- ¼ cup chicken stock
- 1 tablespoon Italian seasoning
- 1 tablespoon parsley, chopped

Directions

1. Heat up a pan with the oil over medium-high heat, add the chicken, garlic, salt and pepper and brown for 3 minutes on each side.
2. Add the rest of the ingredients except the parsley, bring to a simmer and cook over medium-low heat for 40 minutes.
3. Add the parsley, divide the mix between plates and serve.

Nutrition: calories 309; fat 12.4; fiber 11.1; carbs 23.8; protein 15.3

Turkey, Artichokes And Asparagus

Servings: 4 | Cooking: 30 min

Ingredients

- 2 turkey breasts, boneless, skinless and halved
- 3 tablespoons olive oil
- 1 and ½ pounds asparagus, trimmed and halved
- 1 cup chicken stock
- A pinch of salt and black pepper
- 1 cup canned artichoke hearts, drained
- ¼ cup kalamata olives, pitted and sliced
- 1 shallot, chopped
- 3 garlic cloves, minced
- 3 tablespoons dill, chopped

Directions

1. Heat up a pan with the oil over medium-high heat, add the turkey and the garlic and brown for 4 minutes on each side.
2. Add the asparagus, the stock and the rest of the ingredients except the dill, bring to a simmer and cook over medium heat for 20 minutes.

3. Add the dill, divide the mix between plates and serve.

Nutrition: calories 291; fat 16; fiber 10.3; carbs 22.8; protein 34.5

Almond Chicken Bites

Servings: 8 | Cooking: 5 min

Ingredients

- 1-pound chicken fillet
- 1 tablespoon potato starch
- ½ teaspoon salt
- 1 teaspoon paprika
- 2 tablespoons wheat flour, whole grain
- 1 egg, beaten
- 1 tablespoon almond butter

Directions

1. Chop the chicken fillet on the small pieces and place in the bowl.
2. Add egg, salt, and potato starch. Mix up the chicken.
3. Then mix up wheat flour and paprika.
4. Then coat every chicken piece in wheat flour mixture.
5. Place almond butter in the skillet and heat it up.
6. Add chicken popcorn and roast it for 5 minutes over medium heat.

7. Dry the chicken popcorn with the help of the paper towel.

Nutrition: calories 141; fat 5.9; fiber 0.4; carbs 3.3; protein 17.8

Chicken Wings And Dates Mix

Servings: 6 | Cooking: 1 Hour

Ingredients

- 12 chicken wings, halved
- 2 garlic cloves, minced
- Juice of 1 lime
- Zest of 1 lime
- 2 tablespoons avocado oil
- 1 cup dates, pitted and halved
- 1 teaspoon cumin, ground
- Salt and black pepper to the taste
- ½ cup chicken stock
- 1 tablespoon chives, chopped

Directions

1. In a roasting pan, combine the chicken wings with the garlic, lime juice and the rest of the ingredients, toss, introduce in the oven and bake at 360 degrees F for 1 hour.
2. Divide everything between plates and serve with a side salad.

Nutrition: calories 294; fat 19.4; fiber 11.8; carbs 21.4; protein 17.5

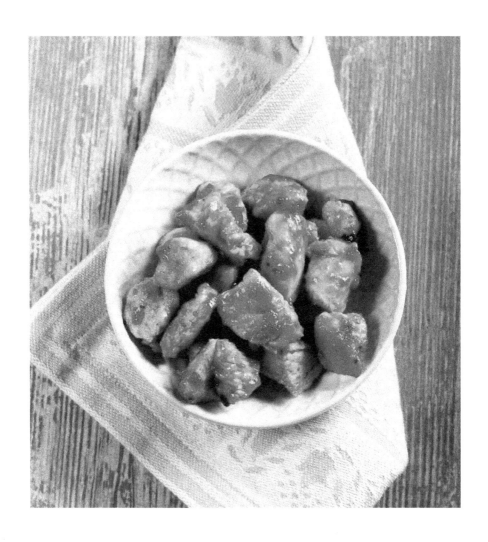

65

Chapter 5: Fish and Seafood Recipes

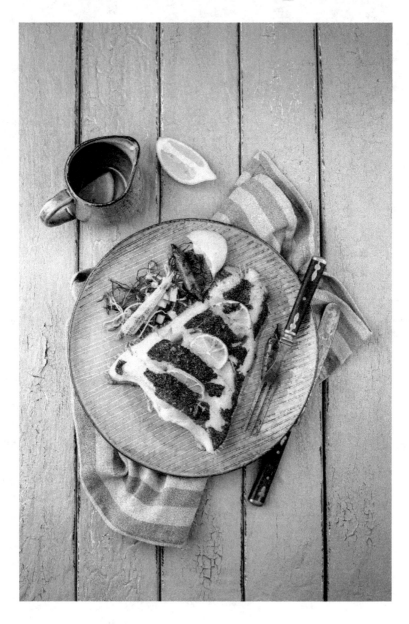

Salmon And Broccoli

Servings: 4 | Cooking: 20 min

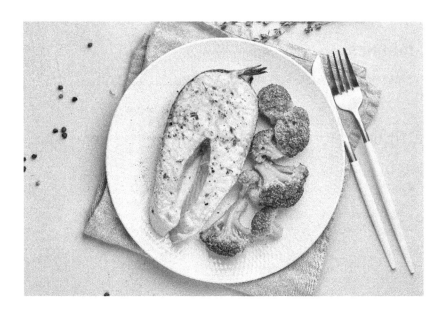

Ingredients

- 2 tablespoons balsamic vinegar
- 1 broccoli head, florets separated
- 4 pieces salmon fillets, skinless
- 1 big red onion, roughly chopped
- 1 tablespoon olive oil
- Sea salt and black pepper to the taste

Directions

1. In a baking dish, combine the salmon with the broccoli and the rest of the ingredients, introduce in the oven and bake at 390 degrees F for 20 minutes.
2. Divide the mix between plates and serve.

Nutrition: calories 302; fat 15.5; fiber 8.5; carbs 18.9; protein 19.8

Halibut And Quinoa Mix

Servings: 4 | Cooking: 12 min

Ingredients

- 4 halibut fillets, boneless
- 2 tablespoons olive oil
- 1 teaspoon rosemary, dried
- 2 teaspoons cumin, ground
- 1 tablespoons coriander, ground
- 2 teaspoons cinnamon powder
- 2 teaspoons oregano, dried
- A pinch of salt and black pepper
- 2 cups quinoa, cooked
- 1 cup cherry tomatoes, halved
- 1 avocado, peeled, pitted and sliced
- 1 cucumber, cubed
- ½ cup black olives, pitted and sliced
- Juice of 1 lemon

Directions

1. In a bowl, combine the fish with the rosemary, cumin, coriander, cinnamon, oregano, salt and pepper and toss.

2. Heat up a pan with the oil over medium heat, add the fish, and sear for 2 minutes on each side.
3. Introduce the pan in the oven and bake the fish at 425 degrees F for 7 minutes.
4. Meanwhile, in a bowl, mix the quinoa with the remaining ingredients, toss and divide between plates.
5. Add the fish next to the quinoa mix and serve right away.

Nutrition: calories 364; fat 15.4; fiber 11.2; carbs 56.4; protein 24.5

Crab Stew

Servings: 2 | Cooking: 13 min

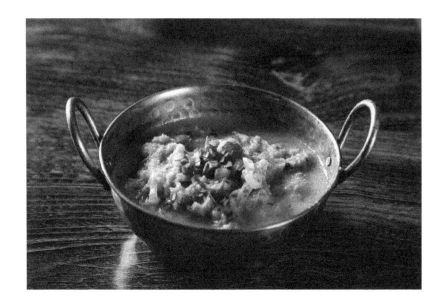

Ingredients

- 1/2 lb lump crab meat
- 2 tbsp heavy cream
- 1 tbsp olive oil
- 2 cups fish stock
- 1/2 lb shrimp, shelled and chopped
- 1 celery stalk, chopped
- 1/2 tsp garlic, chopped
- 1/4 onion, chopped

- Pepper
- Salt

Directions

1. Add oil into the inner pot of instant pot and set the pot on sauté mode.
2. Add onion and sauté for 3 minutes.
3. Add garlic and sauté for 30 seconds.
4. Add remaining ingredients except for heavy cream and stir well.
5. Seal pot with lid and cook on high for 10 minutes.
6. Once done, release pressure using quick release. Remove lid.
7. Stir in heavy cream and serve.

Nutrition: Calories 376 Fat 25.5 g Carbohydrates 5.8 g Sugar 0.7 g Protein 48.1 g Cholesterol 326 mg

Crazy Saganaki Shrimp

Servings: 4 | Cooking: 10 min

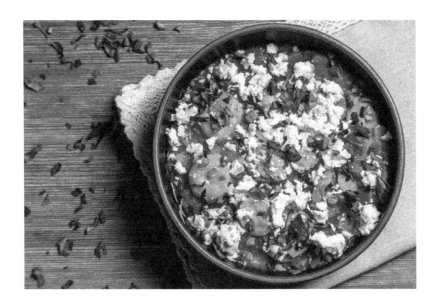

Ingredients

- ¼ tsp salt
- ½ cup Chardonnay
- ½ cup crumbled Greek feta cheese
- 1 medium bulb. fennel, cored and finely chopped
- 1 small Chile pepper, seeded and minced
- 1 tbsp extra virgin olive oil
- 12 jumbo shrimps, peeled and deveined with tails left on

- 2 tbsp lemon juice, divided
- 5 scallions sliced thinly
- Pepper to taste

Directions

1. In medium bowl, mix salt, lemon juice and shrimp.
2. On medium fire, place a saganaki pan (or large nonstick saucepan) and heat oil.
3. Sauté Chile pepper, scallions, and fennel for 4 minutes or until starting to brown and is already soft.
4. Add wine and sauté for another minute.
5. Place shrimps on top of fennel, cover and cook for 4 minutes or until shrimps are pink.
6. Remove just the shrimp and transfer to a plate.
7. Add pepper, feta and 1 tbsp lemon juice to pan and cook for a minute or until cheese begins to melt.
8. To serve, place cheese and fennel mixture on a serving plate and top with shrimps.

Nutrition: Calories per serving: 310; Protein: 49.7g; Fat: 6.8g; Carbs: 8.4g

Grilled Tuna

Servings: 3 | Cooking: 6 min

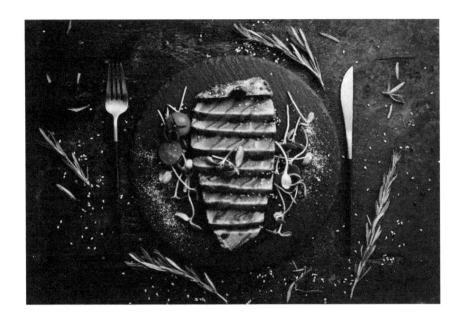

Ingredients

- 3 tuna fillets
- 3 teaspoons teriyaki sauce
- ½ teaspoon minced garlic
- 1 teaspoon olive oil

Directions

1. Whisk together teriyaki sauce, minced garlic, and olive oil.

2. Bruhs every tuna fillet with teriyaki mixture.

3. Preheat grill to 390F.

4. Grill the fish for 3 minutes from each side.

Nutrition: calories 382; fat 32.6; fiber 0; carbs 1.1; protein 21.4

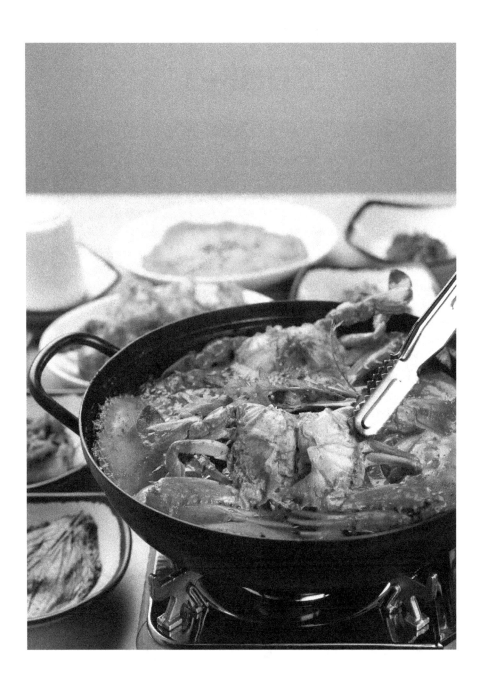

Chapter 6: Salads & Side Dishes

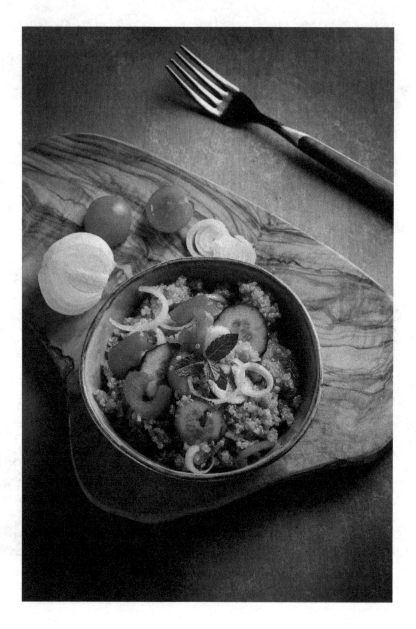

Cucumber Yogurt Gazpacho

Servings: 6 | Cooking: 20 min

Ingredients

- 4 cucumbers, partially peeled
- 1 cup seedless white grapes
- 2 tablespoon sliced almonds
- 1 cup ice cubes
- 2 garlic cloves
- 1 tablespoon chopped dill
- 2 tablespoons cream cheese
- ½ cup plain yogurt
- 2 tablespoons extra virgin olive oil
- Salt and pepper to taste
- 1 tablespoon lemon juice

Directions

1. Combine the cucumbers with the rest of the ingredients in a blender.
2. Add salt and pepper and pulse until smooth and creamy.
3. Serve the gazpacho as fresh as possible.

Nutrition: Calories:111 Fat:7.3g Protein:3.3g
Carbohydrates:9.9g

Creamy Roasted Vegetable Soup

Servings: 8 | Cooking: 45 min

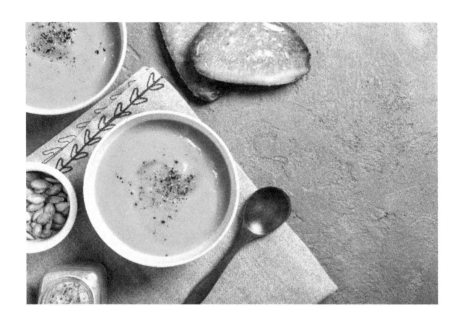

Ingredients

- 2 red onions, sliced
- 1 zucchini, sliced
- 2 tomatoes, sliced
- 2 potatoes, sliced
- 2 garlic cloves
- 2 tablespoons olive oil
- 1 teaspoon dried basil
- 1 teaspoon dried oregano

- 4 cups vegetable stock
- 8 cups water
- Salt and pepper to taste
- 1 bay leaf
- 1 thyme sprig

Directions

1. Combine the onions, zucchini, tomatoes, potatoes, garlic, oil, basil and oregano in a deep dish baking pan.
2. Season with salt and pepper and cook in the preheated oven at 400F for 30 minutes or until golden brown.
3. Transfer the vegetables in a soup pot and add the stock and water.
4. Stir in the bay leaf and thyme sprig and cook for 15 minutes.
5. When done, remove the thyme and bay leaf and puree the soup with an immersion blender.
6. Serve the soup warm and fresh.

Nutrition: Calories:92 Fat:3.8g Protein:2.0g Carbohydrates:13.9g

Turkish Chicken Skewers

Servings: 4 | Cooking: 12 min

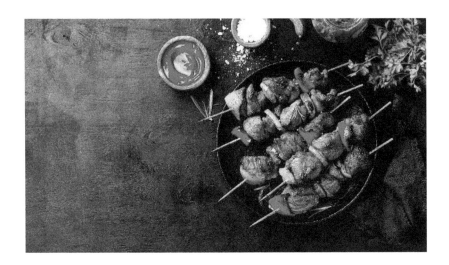

Ingredients

- 2 pounds chicken breasts, boneless skinless, cut into 1 inch cubes
- 2 tablespoons sumac spice, for sprinkling
- 2 lemons, thinly sliced, for skewering
- For the marinade:
- 5 cloves garlic
- 2 roma tomatoes
- 1 lemon, juiced
- 2 tablespoons olive oil
- 1/4 cup yogurt (low fat, full, or fat free)

- 1/4 cup total fresh cilantro and parsley leaves
- 1/2 teaspoon salt
- 1/2 teaspoon pepper
- 1/2 teaspoon allspice
- 1 teaspoon oregano
- 1 teaspoon cinnamon

Directions

1. Preheat the oven to 375F or a grill to medium high heat.
2. Put the marinade ingredients into a food processor; pulse until smooth.
3. Toss the chicken with the marinade. Thread the chicken cubes in skewers, alternating with a thin slice of lemon between chicken cubes.
4. Grill the skewers for about 3-5 minutes per side, covered.
5. When cooked, sprinkle the skewers with generously with the sumac.
6. Serve with plenty of Aryan.

Nutrition:303 cal., 11.1 g total fat (2.1 g sat. fat), 134 mg chol., 247.5 mg sodium, 8 g total carbs., 2.5 g fiber, 2.4 g sugar, 42.5 g protein, 9% vitamin A, 48% vitamin C, 6% calcium, and 9% iron.

Farro with Artichoke Hearts

Preparation: 9 min | Cooking: 41 min | Servings: 6

Ingredients

- 1 cup farro
- 1 bay leaf
- 1 fresh rosemary sprig
- 1 fresh thyme sprig
- 2 tablespoons extra-virgin olive oil
- 1 onion, chopped
- 2 cups frozen artichoke hearts
- 1 tablespoon Italian seasoning
- 3 garlic cloves, minced
- 2 cups unsalted vegetable broth
- Zest of 1 lemon
- ½ teaspoon sea salt
- 1/8 teaspoon freshly ground black pepper
- ¼ cup (about 2 ounces) grated Parmesan cheese

Directions

1. In a medium pot, combine the farro, bay leaf, rosemary, and thyme with enough water to cover it by about 2 inches. Situate it on the stove top over

medium-high heat and bring it to a boil. Set the heat to medium-low and simmer uncovered for 25 to 30 min, stirring occasionally, until the grain is tender. Strain any extra water and set the farro aside. Remove and discard the bay leaf, rosemary, and thyme.

2. Using big skillet over medium-high heat, heat the olive oil until it shimmers.
3. Add the onion, artichoke hearts, and Italian seasoning. Cook for 6 min.
4. Cook the garlic for 30 seconds.
5. Pour in the broth, ½ cup at a time, and stir constantly until the liquid is absorbed before adding the next ½ cup of broth.
6. Stir in the lemon zest, sea salt, pepper, and cheese. Cook for 1 to 2 min more, stirring, until the cheese melts.

Nutrition: Calories: 138; Protein: 7g; Fat: 8g

Vinegar Cucumber Mix

Servings: 6 | Cooking: 0 min

Ingredients

- 1 tablespoon olive oil
- 4 cucumbers, sliced
- Salt and black pepper to the taste
- 1 red onion, chopped
- 3 tablespoons red wine vinegar
- 1 bunch basil, chopped
- 1 teaspoon honey

Directions

1. In a bowl, mix the vinegar with the basil, salt, pepper, the oil and the honey and whisk well.
2. In a bowl, mix the cucumber with the onion and the vinaigrette, toss and serve as a side salad.

Nutrition: calories 182; fat 7.8; fiber 2.1; carbs 4.3; protein 4.1

Garden Salad With Oranges And Olives

Servings: 4 | Cooking: 15 min

Ingredients

- ½ cup red wine vinegar
- 1 tbsp extra virgin olive oil
- 1 tbsp finely chopped celery
- 1 tbsp finely chopped red onion
- 16 large ripe black olives
- 2 garlic cloves
- 2 navel oranges, peeled and segmented
- 4 boneless, skinless chicken breasts, 4-oz each
- 4 garlic cloves, minced
- 8 cups leaf lettuce, washed and dried
- Cracked black pepper to taste

Directions

1. Prepare the dressing by mixing pepper, celery, onion, olive oil, garlic and vinegar in a small bowl. Whisk well to combine.
2. Lightly grease grate and preheat grill to high.

3. Rub chicken with the garlic cloves and discard garlic.
4. Grill chicken for 5 minutes per side or until cooked through.
5. Remove from grill and let it stand for 5 minutes before cutting into ½-inch strips.
6. In 4 serving plates, evenly arrange two cups lettuce, ¼ of the sliced oranges and 4 olives per plate.
7. Top each plate with ¼ serving of grilled chicken, evenly drizzle with dressing, serve and enjoy.

Nutrition: Calories per serving: 259.8; Protein: 48.9g; Carbs: 12.9g; Fat: 1.4g

Mediterranean Garden Salad

Servings: 2 Cups | Cooking: 5 min

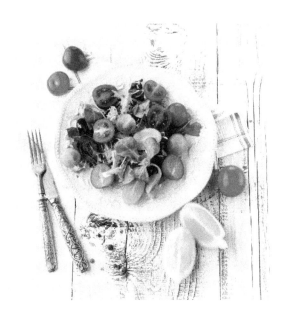

Ingredients

- 6 cups mixed greens
- 2 cups cherry tomatoes, halved
- 1 medium red onion, sliced (1/2 cup)
- 3 TB. tahini paste
- 3 TB. fresh lemon juice
- 3 TB. balsamic vinegar
- 3 TB. plus 1 tsp. extra-virgin olive oil
- 3 TB. water

- 1/2 tsp. salt
- 1/2 tsp. fresh ground black pepper
- 1/2 cup pine nuts

Directions

1. In a large bowl, add mixed greens, cherry tomatoes, and red onion.
2. In a small bowl, whisk together tahini paste, lemon juice, balsamic vinegar, 3 tablespoons extra-virgin olive oil, water, salt, and black pepper.
3. Preheat a small skillet over medium-low heat for 1 minute. Add remaining 1 teaspoon extra-virgin olive oil and pine nuts, and cook, stirring to toast evenly on all sides, for 4 minutes. Transfer pine nuts to a plate, and let cool for 2 minutes.
4. Pour dressing over vegetables, and toss to coat evenly. Top with toasted pine nuts, and serve immediately.

Smoked Salmon Lentil Salad

Servings: 4 | Cooking: 25 min

Ingredients

- 1 cup green lentils, rinsed
- 2 cups vegetable stock
- ½ cup chopped parsley
- 2 tablespoons chopped cilantro
- 1 red pepper, chopped
- 1 red onion, chopped
- Salt and pepper to taste
- 4 oz. smoked salmon, shredded
- 1 lemon, juiced

Directions

1. Combine the lentils and stock in a saucepan. Cook on low heat for 15-20 minutes or until all the liquid has been absorbed completely.
2. Transfer the lentils in a salad bowl and add the parsley, cilantro, red pepper and onion. Season with salt and pepper.
3. Add the smoked salmon and lemon juice and mix well.

4. Serve the salad fresh.

Nutrition: Calories:233 Fat:2.0g Protein:18.7g
Carbohydrates:35.5g

Salmon & Arugula Salad

Servings: 2 | Cooking: 12 min

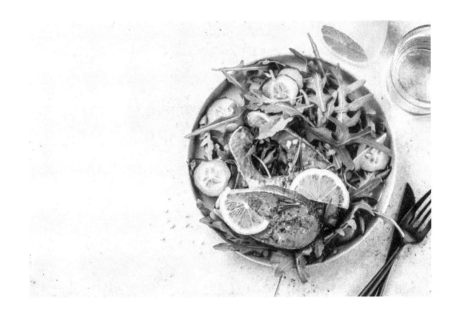

Ingredients

- ¼ cup red onion, sliced thinly
- 1 ½ tbsp fresh lemon juice
- 1 ½ tbsp olive oil
- 1 tbsp extra-virgin olive oil
- 1 tbsp red-wine vinegar
- 2 center cut salmon fillets (6-oz each)
- 2/3 cup cherry tomatoes, halved
- 3 cups baby arugula leaves

- Pepper and salt to taste

Directions

1. In a shallow bowl, mix pepper, salt, 1 ½ tbsp olive oil and lemon juice. Toss in salmon fillets and rub with the marinade. Allow to marinate for at least 15 minutes.
2. Grease a baking sheet and preheat oven to 3500F.
3. Bake marinated salmon fillet for 10 to 12 minutes or until flaky with skin side touching the baking sheet.
4. Meanwhile, in a salad bowl mix onion, tomatoes and arugula.
5. Season with pepper and salt. Drizzle with vinegar and oil. Toss to combine and serve right away with baked salmon on the side.

Nutrition: Calories per serving: 400; Protein: 36.6g; Carbs: 5.8g; Fat: 25.6g

Keto Bbq Chicken Pizza Soup

Servings: 6 | Cooking: 1 Hour 30 min

Ingredients

- 6 chicken legs
- 1 medium red onion, diced
- 4 garlic cloves
- 1 large tomato, unsweetened
- 4 cups green beans
- ¾ cup BBQ Sauce
- 1½ cups mozzarella cheese, shredded
- ¼ cup ghee
- 2 quarts water
- 2 quarts chicken stock
- Salt and black pepper, to taste
- Fresh cilantro, for garnishing

Directions

1. Put chicken, water and salt in a large pot and bring to a boil.
2. Reduce the heat to medium-low and cook for about 75 minutes.

3. Shred the meat off the bones using a fork and keep aside.
4. Put ghee, red onions and garlic in a large soup and cook over a medium heat.
5. Add chicken stock and bring to a boil over a high heat.
6. Add green beans and tomato to the pot and cook for about 15 minutes.
7. AddBBQ Sauce, shredded chicken, salt and black pepper to the pot.
8. Ladle the soup into serving bowls and top with shredded mozzarella cheese and cilantro to serve.

Nutrition: Calories: 449 Carbs: 7.1g Fats: 32.5g Proteins: 30.8g Sodium: 252mg Sugar: 4.7g

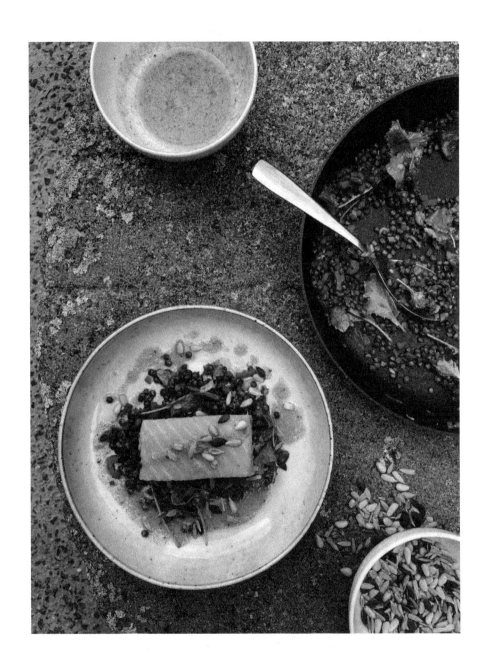

Chapter 7: Dessert Recipes

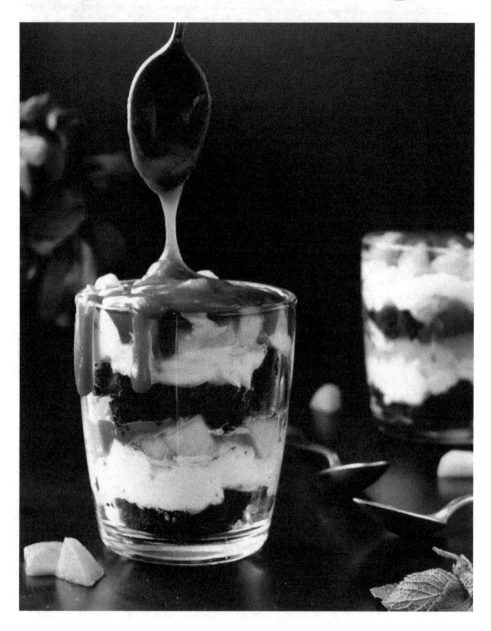

White Wine Grapefruit Poached Peaches

Servings: 6 | Cooking: 40 min

Ingredients

- 4 peaches
- 2 cups white wine
- 1 grapefruit, peeled and juiced
- ¼ cup white sugar
- 1 cinnamon stick
- 1 star anise
- 1 cardamom pod
- 1 cup Greek yogurt for serving

Directions

1. Combine the wine, grapefruit, sugar and spices in a saucepan.
2. Bring to a boil then place the peaches in the hot syrup.
3. Lower the heat and cover with a lid. Cook for 15 minutes then allow to cool down.
4. Carefully peel the peaches and place them in a small serving bowl.

5. Top with yogurt and serve right away.

Nutrition: Calories:157 Fat:0.9g Protein:4.2g
Carbohydrates:20.4g

Cinnamon Stuffed Peaches

Servings: 4 | Cooking: 5 min

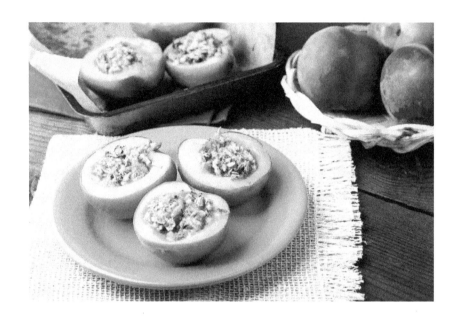

Ingredients

- 4 peaches, pitted, halved
- 2 tablespoons ricotta cheese
- 2 tablespoons of liquid honey
- ¾ cup of water
- ½ teaspoon vanilla extract
- ¾ teaspoon ground cinnamon
- 1 tablespoon almonds, sliced
- ¾ teaspoon saffron

Directions

1. Pour water in the saucepan and bring to boil.
2. Add vanilla extract, saffron, ground cinnamon, and liquid honey.
3. Cook the liquid until the honey is melted.
4. Then remove it from the heat.
5. Put the halved peaches in the hot honey liquid.
6. Meanwhile, make the filling: mix up together ricotta cheese, vanilla extract, and sliced almonds.
7. Remove the peaches from honey liquid and arrange in the plate.
8. Fill 4 peach halves with ricotta filling and cover them with remaining peach halves.
9. Sprinkle the cooked dessert with liquid honey mixture gently.

Nutrition: calories 113; fat 1.8; fiber 2.8; carbs 23.9; protein 2.7

Eggless Farina Cake (namoura)

Servings: 1 Piece | Cooking: 40 min

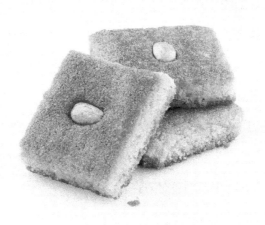

Ingredients

- 2 cups farina
- 1/2 cup semolina
- 1/2 cup all-purpose flour
- 1 TB. baking powder
- 1 tsp. active dry yeast
- 1/2 cup sugar
- 1/2 cup plain Greek yogurt
- 1 cup whole milk

- 3/4 cup butter, melted
- 1/4 cup water
- 2 TB. tahini paste
- 15 almonds
- 2 cups Simple Syrup

Directions

1. In a large bowl, combine farina, semolina, all-purpose flour, baking powder, yeast, sugar, Greek yogurt, whole milk, butter, and water. Set aside for 15 minutes.

2. Preheat the oven to 375°F.

3. Spread tahini paste evenly in the bottom of a 9×13-inch baking pan, and pour in cake batter. Arrange almonds on top of batter, about where each slice will be. Bake for 45 minutes or until golden brown.

4. Remove cake from the oven, and using a toothpick, poke holes throughout cake for Simple Syrup to seep into. Pour syrup over cake, and let cake sit for 1 hour to absorb syrup.

5. Cool cake completely before cutting and serving.

Banana And Berries Trifle

Servings: 10 | Cooking: 5 min

Ingredients

- 8 oz biscuits, chopped
- ¼ cup strawberries, chopped
- 1 banana, chopped
- 1 peach, chopped
- ½ mango, chopped
- 1 cup grapes, chopped
- 1 tablespoon liquid honey
- 1 cup of orange juice
- ½ cup Plain yogurt
- ¼ cup cream cheese
- 1 teaspoon coconut flakes

Directions

1. Bring the orange juice to boil and remove it from the heat.
2. Add liquid honey and stir until it is dissolved.
3. Cool the liquid to the room temperature.

4. Add chopped banana, peach, mango, grapes, and strawberries. Shake the fruits gently and leave to soak the orange juice for 15 minutes.
5. Meanwhile, with the help of the hand mixer mix up together Plain yogurt and cream cheese.
6. Then separate the chopped biscuits, yogurt mixture, and fruits on 4 parts.
7. Place the first part of biscuits in the big serving glass in one layer.
8. Spread it with yogurt mixture and add fruits.
9. Repeat the same steps till you use all ingredients.
10. Top the trifle with coconut flakes.

Nutrition: calories 164; fat 6.2; fiber 1.3; carbs 24.8; protein 3.2

Mixed Berry Sorbet

Servings: 8 | Cooking: 2 ½ Hours

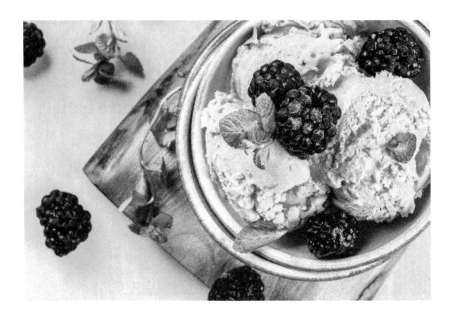

Ingredients

- 2 cups water
- ½ cup white sugar
- 2 cups mixed berries
- 1 tablespoon lemon juice
- 2 tablespoons honey
- 1 teaspoon lemon zest
- 1 mint sprig

Directions

1. Combine the water, sugar, berries, lemon juice, honey and lemon zest in a saucepan.
2. Bring to a boil and cook on low heat for 5 minutes.
3. Add the mint sprig and remove off heat. Allow to infuse for 10 minutes then remove the mint.
4. Pour the syrup into a blender and puree until smooth and creamy.
5. Pour the smooth syrup into an airtight container and freeze for at least 2 hours.
6. Serve the sorbet chilled.

Nutrition: Calories:84 Fat:0.1g Protein:0.4g Carbohydrates:21.3g

CPSIA information can be obtained
at www.ICGtesting.com
Printed in the USA
LVHW081519120621
690063LV00003B/187

9 781911 688884